SINGL[illegible]
SUR[illegible]OR

Sharon Rose

ARTHUR H. STOCKWELL LTD
Torrs Park Ilfracombe Devon
Established 1898
www.ahstockwell.co.uk

First published in Great Britain, 2010

British Library Cataloguing-in-Publication Data.
A catalogue record for this book is available from the British Library.

ISBN 978-0-7223-4004-2
Printed in Great Britain by
Arthur H. Stockwell Ltd
Torrs Park Ilfracombe
Devon

DEDICATION

I dedicate this book to my family and friends because without them there wouldn't be a story.

Without affection for all of them, there wouldn't be any substance to the story.

Donations from royalties of book sales will be made to Cancer Research UK.

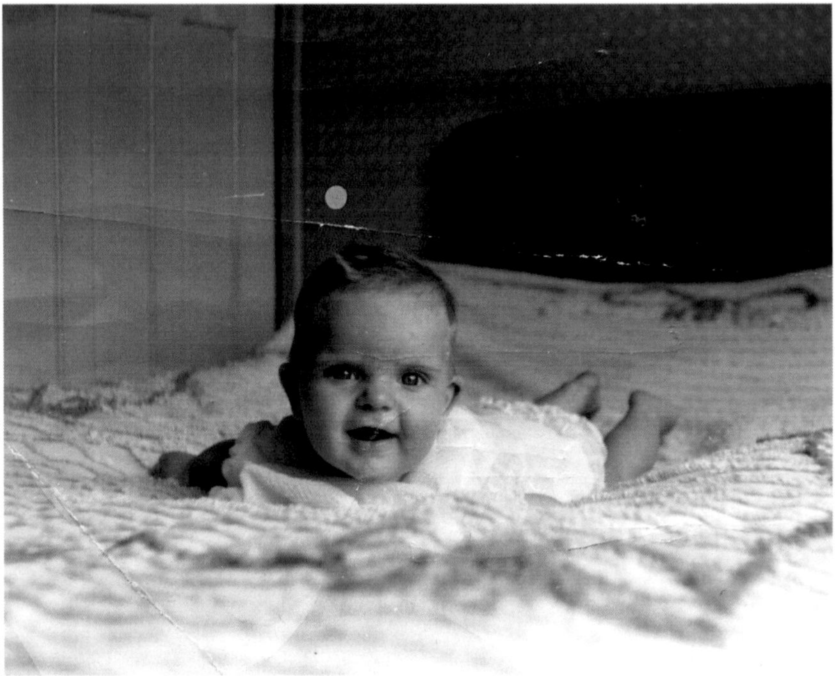

Me as a baby, 1960.

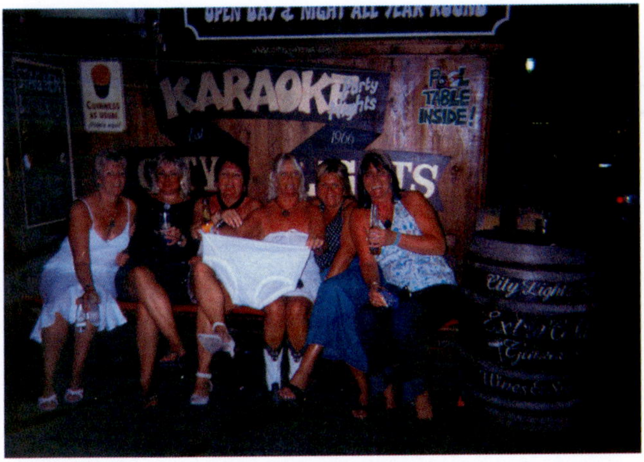

Magaluf, 2005.

Magaluf, September 2005

My life was hunky-dory. I had fulfilled my career aspirations, ended another failed marriage, found a passion in salsa dancing, and formed a strong network of new friends. I was on a soft, sandy beach in the hot sunshine on my first girly holiday. I looked at the sea and thought, 'Things are going too well for me.' I sensed something was waiting for me around the next corner of life.

And it was.

My social life was buzzing, and I looked and felt my best in years. People stopped me in the street and commented on how well I looked. But I was walking around with cancer and didn't know it.

I was in the shower when I found it, as clear and defined as could be: a lump in my right breast. No matter how I stood or lay down, that lump did not go away. Friends tried to reassure me: they said it was bound to be a cyst.

But I knew different. I just knew it was breast cancer.

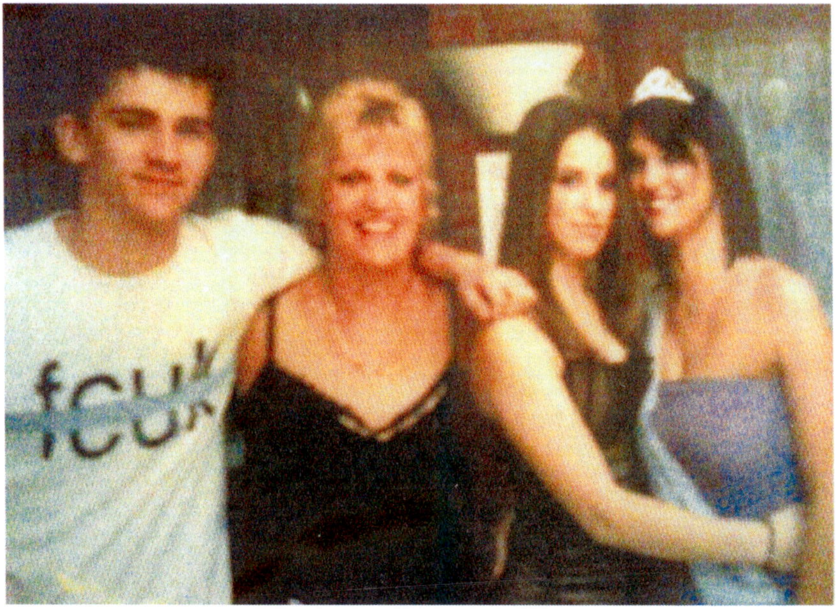

My son, Alistair, Me, and my two daughters, Lisa and Fiona.

October 2005

I had so much to look forward to. Both my daughters had such a busy month. It was Fiona's twenty-first and Lisa was dancing with the National Youth Ballet in Sevenoaks in Kent and London's Drury Lane. I wanted all these lovely things out of the way before I dropped the bombshell. Eventually I went to the doctors, and initially the GP thought it was nothing to worry about. For a week I wanted to believe her, but instinct told me to go back.

I waited only two weeks to go to the breast clinic.

My life was about to change, physically, emotionally and spiritually, for my mum, my sister, my children, my best friends and, most of all, for **ME**!

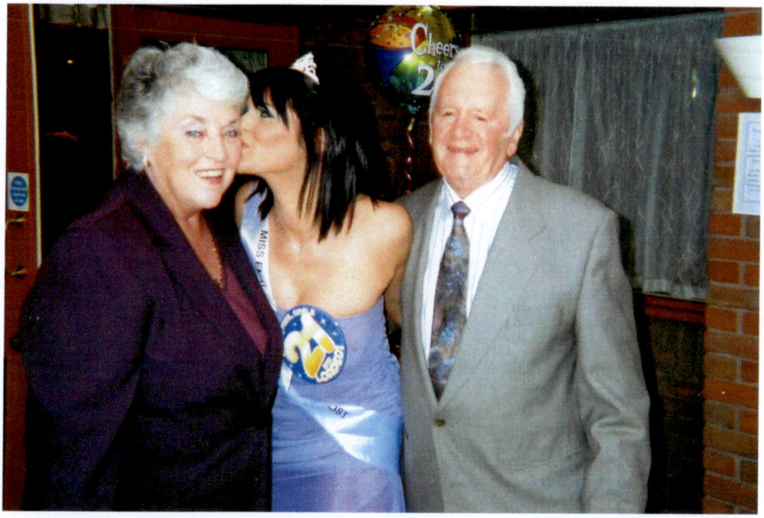

My mum and stepdad (Mike) on Fiona's 21st birthday, October 2005.

The Roller-Coaster Ride, 28 November 2005

I will never forget this day. The consultant was pretty confident it was not cancer and off I went for a mammogram, but in the X-ray department there was suddenly an aura of impending doom. I could see by their faces and read in their smiles that the news was not going to be good. I cried when the doctor took the biopsies, especially as I had two lumps and I hadn't even noticed the other one. I cried at this stage – not because it hurt, but because I was now frightened.

I didn't cry in front of my mum, sister (Helen) and best friend (Janine). They were shocked and upset, and we all left the hospital in disbelief, apprehensive about what was to happen next.

30 November 2005

The diagnosis of lobular breast cancer was confirmed. It was explained to me that this is a fast-spreading cancer of the breast tissue and surgery would involve a right mastectomy and removal of lymph nodes.

I was given the option of breast reconstruction, but this would have delayed my mastectomy. I just wanted the cancer out of my body and the breast removed.

December 2005

I had waited for seven days to go into hospital, and in that time I had the strangest experiences and lived life to the full. I didn't think for one minute the man I had been seeing for the previous months would say goodbye on the day I went into hospital, but that is what happened. I haven't seen him or heard from him since.

I am not frightened of dying – not any more – but I was cursing at times in hospital. God got the blame, and I kept saying, "If my time's up, stop prolonging the agony."

The random contradiction of a mind in turmoil.

The hospital experience was a mixture of sadness, laughter, fear and pain. Whilst I was in hospital having my mastectomy, friends and family brought magazines; but I couldn't concentrate at all. I verged on mania as I tried to stop myself thinking of the prospect of dying.

Graham, a friend and one of my salsa dancing partners, came sweeping in like a knight in shining armour, with a card, chocolates and flowers. My fellow patients were very impressed. They thought he was my fiancé – and if not, he *should* be!

Salsa tune: 'Lady'.

A patient with spiritual connections said Graham was going to be more to me than a friend, and she was right. Her premonitions gave me the heebie-jeebies. I decided it was time to for me to go home.

My son, Alistair, asked me when I was going home, and I knew it was important for me to get home for Christmas. I went home on 20 December 2005

My homecoming was very emotional. My family had decorated a real Christmas tree for me, and I cried. I didn't think I would see Christmas again.

I have always been a positive-thinking person, but now I was on 'cancer planet'. I am still a positive person, but I found it hard to come to terms with what I was going to be put through.

I now live for the day and never discuss my retirement plans.

I didn't want to know the results from the surgical biopsy because if the news was bad, I couldn't think of anything worse for myself and my family – especially just before Christmas.

The specialist breast-care nurse asked me why I didn't want to know the results. She said, "What if the results are fairly positive, with grade-2 cancer and no lymph-node involvement?"

I hugged her and said you have given me the best Christmas present ever: **HOPE**.

On Christmas Eve I treated myself to a wig. I had always wanted long blonde hair, so I thought, 'Let's go for it! It was the strangest Christmas present I had bought myself ever.

New Year's Eve is always a time when, as a singleton,

there only seem to be couples in the world except for you – your on-your-own, single self. This year I was just glad to be alive and amongst friends. Being single was the last of my worries, and being part of a couple again sadly seemed a dream of the past.

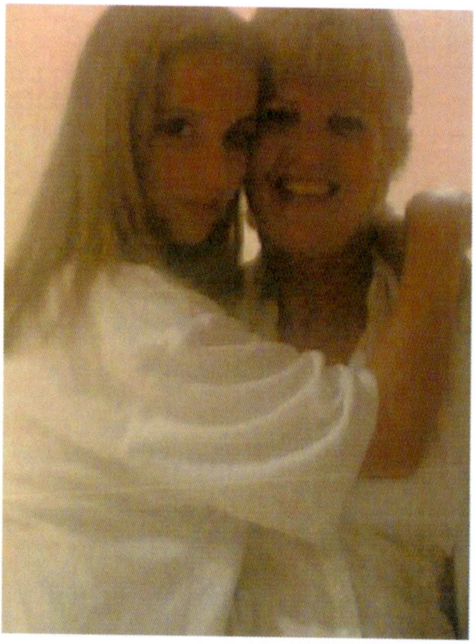

Me and Lisa, after breast surgery.

The Hickman Line

I was frightened and cried my eyes out.

My consultant couldn't believe it. He said, "But you had major surgery two weeks ago and you didn't shed a tear."

It was the thought of it going into the vein in my heart! It freaked me out. I had a sedative and didn't feel a thing for the rest of my treatment. I just had to take care of my Hickman line to prevent any complications: having shallow baths instead of showers, cleaning my hands regularly with antibacterial hand gel and weekly dressings at the hospital. I never had a blocked Hickman line because I danced salsa the night before my chemotherapy, and I think my twizzling kept the line clear.

Chemotherapy

The day came to discuss the chemotherapy regime with the oncologist. I remember sitting there waiting to be called and I watched as women with no hair but wearing scarves and wigs wandered around with drip stands, wonder drugs running through their veins. They were pale and drawn, enduring chemotherapy in the hope that the lurking cancer cells would be destroyed.

It hit me like a thunderbolt: *I had cancer*.

I ran out of the ward to get some fresh air and regain some control and sanity at the same time. I telephoned a friend of mine, Phil. He had been there every day in the hospital, but I was beginning to rely on his support too much. It may have been irrational, but I asked him to step back and not give me the false hope of thinking he would always be there for me. Now it was time to go it alone. I walked back into the ward with the knowledge that there was not going to be a partner to hold me when times were bad during the long, gruelling months of my illness.

On 26th January 2006, I had my first chemotherapy. The massive dose of steroids made my bum tingle as they administered it. (What was that all about!) The chemo takes about forty minutes to administer using the Hickman line. Wham!

For the first three days afterwards I was as high as a kite.

I went to Blackpool on a salsa weekend after my first chemo. It coincided with my good week on the chemotherapy, and I stayed out late and danced all night. When I came home I had a bad cold. My neutrophils were down, meaning my resistance to infection was low, and I started antibiotics straight away. I realised that I had to be sensible in retaining normality. Instead I had to focus on self-preservation. This experience made me aware of the risk of infection whilst having chemotherapy.

I awoke one morning and hair was all over my pillow. When I ran my hands through my hair, I pulled out clumps of it. I couldn't see the point in extending the agony, so I went to the hairdresser with a cap ready to put on after the deed had been done. I asked her to shave it all off.

She was so kind, but later she told me it really upset her. I wasn't upset about losing my hair: it was part of the process to my recovery. A big tub of Vaseline from the Pound Shop is an essential. If it is good enough for babies' bottoms, it was good enough for my head, my eyebrow line and spiky eyelashes. I rubbed the Vaseline daily into my bald head, and I think it helped my hair grow back quickly. It was really soft, curly and black when it did grow back – like duck feathers.

Chemo affects people in different ways. My main problem was gastric pain and constipation. At times I couldn't move to get a drink. I wallowed in the peace of darkness, and emotionally I fell into a black hole. I wanted to revisit my past and to be once again myself, Shazza, a person with confidence and high self-esteem, healthy and beautiful outside. All areas of my life had been moving in a positive direction. I had a future. I had until recently worked as a manager, and I felt proud that I had achieved this position in my career. I had a reasonable salary and I lived in a nice apartment.

I had been able to help and support my children and felt I was no longer a victim of two failed marriages. But now I had cancer. I was lifeless.

I craved strawberries, orange juice, Smash potatoes, coconut cake, chips and mayo, and cherry muffins; and when I had that seven-day normal week with a normal, everyday appetite I would eat a big, yummy bacon-and-mushroom sandwich.

I was grieving for my 'mortality'. The jokes, the denial, the brave face were an act – all part of my strategy of survival. At times I was tempted to allow myself to fall down the black hole for the duration of the treatment, but that thought never lasted long. What a waste of life that would have been! Instead I would get out of bed, put on my make-up, my long blonde wig, my smartest clothes and walk, head held high, with the most essential thing in life – a smile.

I couldn't see properly (my vision was blurred) and my balance was poor, but inside my head is a strength and positive energy that drove me to carry on to live for my children.

I still can't talk about them without crying.

28 February 2006

For forty-five years I had taken my birthday for granted, but in 2006 I greeted the day with a feeling of indescribable elation. Cancer patients have heightened sensory perception: every raindrop that falls on your face, every snowflake or ray of bright sunshine, touches your soul and makes you realise how grateful you are to be alive. *Superficial* is no longer in my dictionary; emotionally I am unsuited to living in the 'single' world and taking part in superficial dating games – not now.

Grieving for the loss of your 'mortality' creeps up on you again further down the line. When treatment is over and friends and family return to the planet of life, you remain on 'cancer planet' asking for a while, "Why me?" Having spent time planning for your demise, you slowly find you are asked to make plans for the future, and it takes time before you feel safe enough to jump back to the planet of life.

The Charity Disco, 3 March 2006

I had to have all my friends under the same roof, and, never one to miss out on a party, I arranged a 'pre-wake' party. I raised £750 that night for charities close to my heart. (A friend and colleague had lung cancer.)

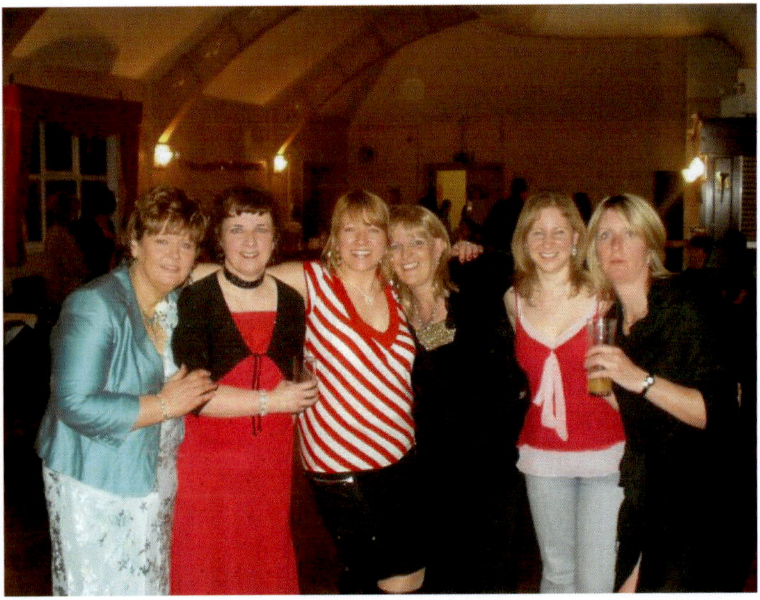

My salsa friends who supported me, at my charity disco, 2006.

March 2006

When I was down, sometimes I would dance around my flat to a record of Andy Abraham singing 'I Love You, Baby'. I loved listening to music. It compensated for not being able to concentrate on reading.

When I was frightened I would sleep at my lovely neighbour's flat. Steve was my karmic soulmate and he said he would never let me die alone. His brother, Bob, used to play the guitar to relax me. He was very spiritual was Bob.

The chemo was kicking in. When I looked in the mirror, I thought, 'Oh, my God, Sharon, you look like a chemo patient! And then I looked again and said to myself, "You *are* a chemo patient."

I had a pain in my right side again. I was frightened that cancer was somewhere else in my body.

One Sunday – the worst day of the week – I wondered if I would feel closer to God now that I had cancer, so I walked into the most beautiful church in Tamworth. However, despite its beauty I felt more at home with my faith in the Catholic church. On the other hand, I have an eclectic approach to religion; I do believe in the positivity of the higher self, and I can be very spiritual at times.

I was craving love and affection. I wanted to be held.

Single with cancer, a double-edged sword:
Nobody else's feelings to consider
But no one to share your world.
'Make sure you are a priority' –
Well, that's a laugh, you see.
Parenting doesn't finish
When you are diagnosed with the big C.

The middle of the night when darkness falls
And you lie alone in silence –
Sometimes the silence is welcomed,
And sometimes you wish it would cease.
Then a new day arrives
And you are pleased to see it here,
For when you are diagnosed with cancer
Every day is a precious year.

I was on my fourth dose of epirubicin and the chemo feeling had kicked in. My worst side effects were constipation and excruciating gastric pain. I was also taking lansoprazole tablets, movicol sachets and orange juice. I had not had any sickness, although the steroids made me look a bit like a sumo wrestler.

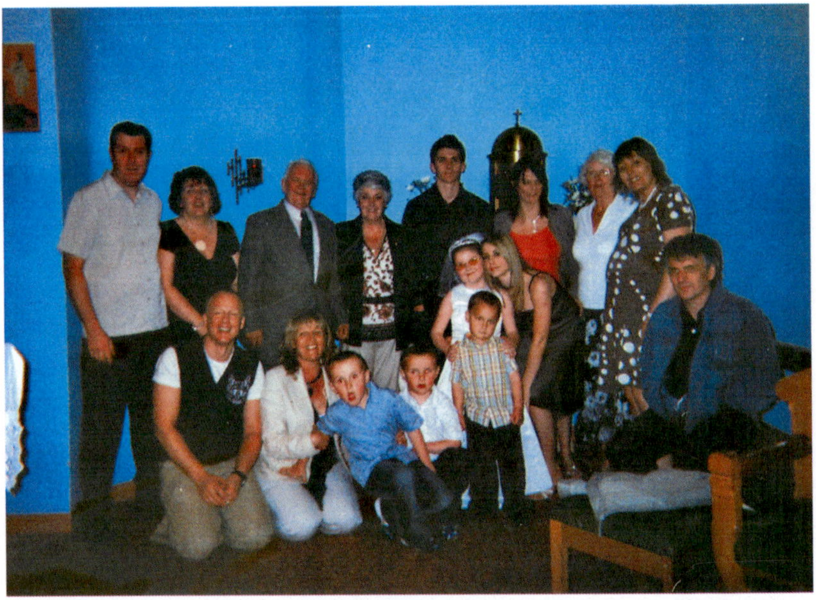

Family photo at my niece Sophie's Holy Communion.

Self-Esteem

I went for an interview, gave a presentation and had very positive feedback. Even though I didn't get the job, I still had brain cells that hadn't been frazzled by chemotherapy. I felt so good about myself! I had had contact with some normality. Stressful as it was to get back in touch with my job, I missed my role as service manager and the daily work challenges that went with it – but now life itself was a challenge.

I tell the important people in my life how much I care for them. Somehow my life is more enriched.

Friendship

Sometimes in difficult situations friends come out of the woodwork and support you all the way. Others stay away from you; only they know why.

Long-lasting friendship is not to do with empty words, it is about showing you care with actions and mutual respect for each other. Friends are people you have a connection with, male or female. In my case, this means they should laugh at my jokes; and my single female friends should never fancy the same men as I do.

I say to my friends, "Value your partner. Don't moan about trivia."

My favourite film is *Shall We Dance?* with Jennifer Lopez and Richard Gere.

My favourite line from the film is, "*Your life will not go unnoticed because I will notice it. Your life will not go unwitnessed because I will be your witness.*"

My friends helped me through the scary journey of cancer. I couldn't have done it without them.

I had only known Jill since July 2005, when we met at our first night at salsa, but we became almost inseparable. We even slept together in a big bed, but we made sure people knew we did not fancy each other!

Jill cared for me on my worse weekends of chemo. She kept me laughing and strong during times when otherwise I would have rolled about in agony. I even had my own chemo toilet at her house. (I think I might have been to blame for the plumbing problems.) Toilet humour was a focus as constipation was my main problem. I did not need to take any anti-sickness pills, which just shows how chemotherapy affects different people in different ways.

Jill and I are oddballs. Our behaviour was totally random and most inappropriate, in the most serious of circumstance.

One Tuesday I was late for chemo club, and we had to rush off with 'bump and grind' blaring out of the CD player. We took our tea and toast in the car to ensure we got to chemo club on time.

We used to have fun with the nurses – especially about my love antics. I was told that I must wear a condom if having sex, to protect myself from infection of any kind and as there was also a slight risk of chemo transferring to the male during intercourse. That prompted jokes about my boyfriends leaving the flat with a baldhead.

All my friends have different qualities. Janine has been my loyal, true, wonderful friend since the age of eleven. We have been each other's bridesmaids (in my case twice) and godmothers to each other's children (and in my case, I am known as Rock Mother). Our friendship is unconditional – and that includes her children and her husband, Ian. My cancer devastated her, I know, and I would have felt the same if it had happened to her. I asked her to come to chemo with me, but it really upset her. I understood. I told her it was OK to cry. She told me off for laughing and said, "If you say you are fine one more time, I'm going to go mad."

One time, when we came out of chemo club, I was laughing and joking, but Janine could not stop crying. Laughter was my way of dealing with things.

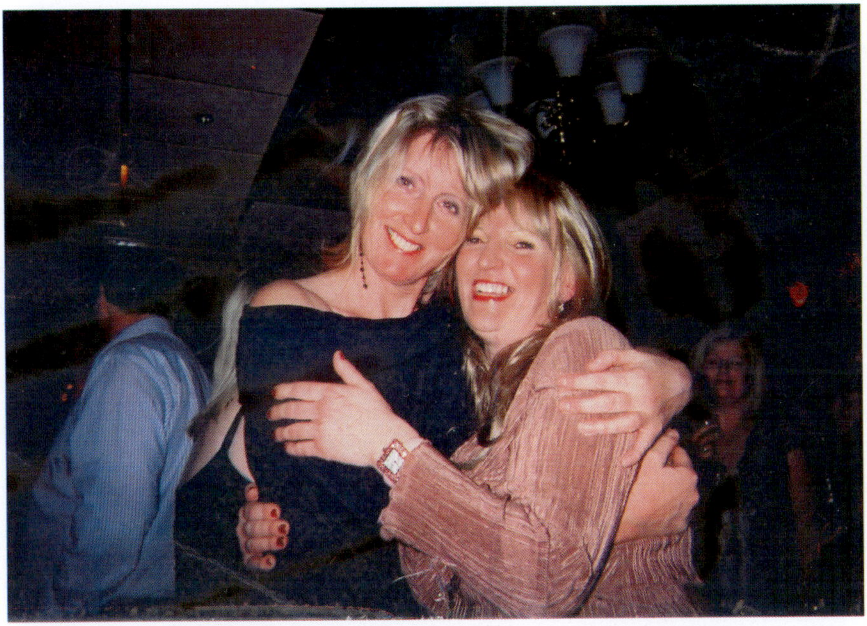

Me and Jill at a charity disco, march 2006.

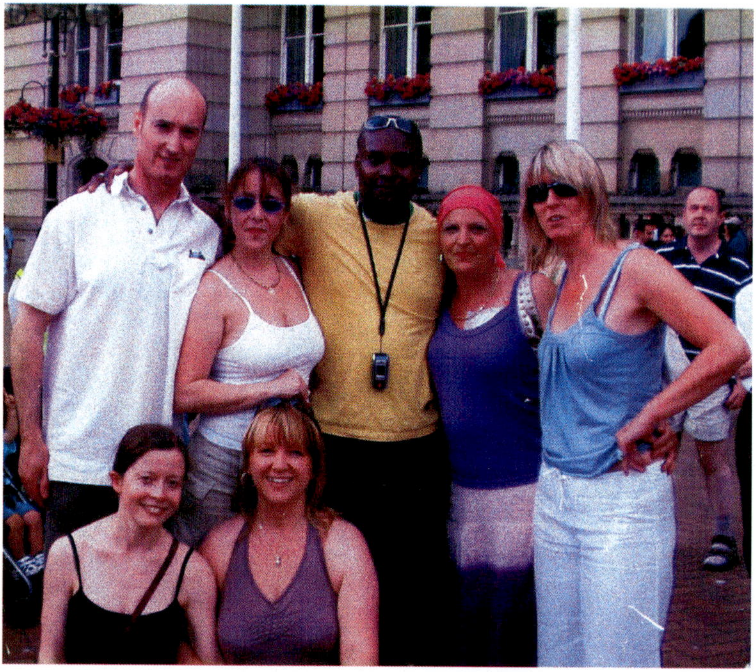

Salsa friends at the Salsa Festival,
Birmingham, summer 2006.

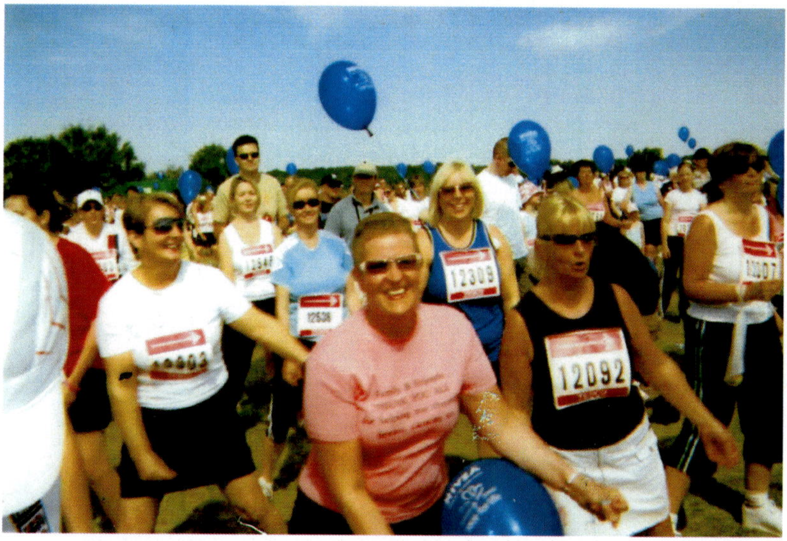

Doing the Race for Life with Lynn and friends, summer 2006.

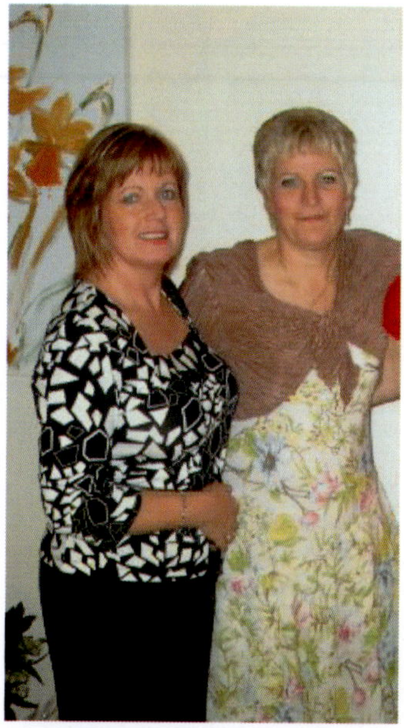

Hidden pain of radiotherapy: with Marion at Hoar Cross Hall, October 2006.

Anger !

I am *bleep* angry! I didn't want to have cancer and to have *bleep* chemotherapy pumped round my *bleep* body. I hated the *bleep* uncertainty of life and not knowing whether I was going to be there for my kids. I wanted to go back to the world of stressing out over minor mishaps. I felt *bleep* alone in the world. What did I do to *bleep* deserve this? I had spent so many years caring for others, and my reward was to have my life cut short by *bleep* cancer.

I was going *bleep* mad in those four walls, but I didn't feel well enough to get out. I was cross. I felt sick and weak and I had that *bleep* pain in my right side again. I was ANGRY, ANGRY, ANGRY!

7 April 2006

I felt better. That night I was to going to salsa to be with friends, and, however ill I felt, I was determined to dance, dance and dance! I would sometimes say, "I will take my salsa shoes just in case." Then I'd be found dancing all night.

The children thing was still not resolved.

I noticed a swelling in my neck. I was scared. I telephoned for advice and had to go in. Was it secondaries or a blood clot?

What ever happened to the common cold – the simple things in life? Cancer is such a reality check. Sometimes I avoided the fact that I had a serious illness; and sometimes I prayed, "Don't take my life away yet." I had just learnt about the real me, the new me, the person who was going to put herself first for a change and live life to the full.

I looked like an alien. Three more chemos to go. Hurray! I couldn't wait to get my hair back, get the Hickman line out and get on with radiotherapy.

I didn't want to die, but I thought about how my children would feel if I did. I didn't want them to grieve for too long or feel sorry that my life was cut short or that my life had been bad. Yes, I have had challenges but actually I have had a fantastic life. Every day I loved going to work as a nurse. I have met wonderful people on my way. In my opinion, mental illness is worse than cancer. My poor dad has suffered all his life with schizophrenia, and he has been under psychiatric care since the age of thirty-nine – but that's another story.

Cakes and Celebrations, July 2006

My last chemo was on 13 July, and my decree absolute came through on 11 July. I am a divorced woman.

Fiona, Alistair, my mum, Jill (my friend from salsa) and Helen (my sister) all piled into the chemotherapy ward. We took a cake and balloons for the patients and the nurses. I was celebrating my last chemo. What I failed to see at first was the woman crying. When I did see her, I asked her why she was crying.

She said, "My cancer has come back and I am going to die, I know I am."

I said to her, "Not today you're not, and any one of us in this room could die tomorrow."

She smiled and I walked away feeling a bit guilty about my joviality, but that is how I cope with things. I make the best of the worst scenario.

I felt humble. My workmates, friends and family had all pulled together to help me and do nice things for me. You need that if you are a single parent living on your own. The children did not have the emotional maturity or logical resource to help me. They appeared to be in denial, and sometimes this drove me mad. We usually argued around the time I felt my worst after the chemotherapy.

I appeared to have a strange bluish-grey skin tone, and my head felt as though it was going to come off my shoulders.

I went to salsa and was very, very chemo'd and wobbly. The men at salsa were so kind. They still danced with me, holding me up as I twizzled around disorientated. What I loved most of all was looking around at all the happy faces enjoying themselves – enjoying life. It was so infectious.

The Children

My heart is divided into six parts – one for each child, one reserved for Erica, my grandchild, one for my closest family and dearest friends, and one reserved for a possible future partner.

They are equal parts, but they have different expressions and emotions. A mother's love for a child is the deepest emotion a soul can carry.

I love my children. My life has been enriched by them. Every single day I have looked into their faces, listened to their voices and watched them grow. I am so proud of them! Every football match, dance routine and singing on stage has given me a lifetime of pleasure.

If I cry when I mention my children, so be it.

"The greatest love of all." (Andy Abraham)

The Hidden Pain of Radiotherapy

I was emotional on my first visit to the Cancer Unit for assessment for radiotherapy. I had the Cancer Unit in my face every day for fifteen days. The unit should be called the 'I Am Glad to Be Alive' unit.

They took X-rays and I was frightened that they would find that the cancer had spread to my lungs. I stared at their faces, trying to pick up any signs of empathy whenever they looked in my direction. They lined me up ready for each X-ray and warned me not to move.

My friend Marion had not seen me cry before, but I couldn't stop. She ferried me out to the car as soon as we could get away.

Before the start of the course I underestimated the effects of radiotherapy. The therapy itself does not hurt at all, but, as those rays are infiltrating the body, energy just drains out of you. The reaction is more or less immediate, and I personally think the resulting tiredness is a permanent fixture.

I nurtured my skin with E45 cream. It stopped irritation and soreness. I washed with Simple soap and used no deodorant.

When I lay still on the table it was the first time I had stayed still in eight months. I had always kept busy and active to stop myself from thinking about cancer and to test my fitness levels and stamina. The tears rolled down my face slowly – controlled crying because I couldn't sob. It was a chance to cry in private for fifteen minutes, but even this short time was too long to be alone with my thoughts.

After radiotherapy you are advised that you may be prone to fractured ribs as the chest wall is weakened. There may also be a residual cough. These side effects are a small price to pay.

23 July 2006

I felt dreadful. There was nobody around at weekends; so if I was terminally ill, I knew I would have to go into a hospice. Everyone has their own life at weekends.

I hate Sundays.

At this time I couldn't see much point in my life. I felt so alone. Life was boring. I thought, 'What's the use? The children only want me for my pension. What's the use? I will die and be forgotten in a few months' time.'

2 August 2006

I had been very emotional lately. I had no money and I had moved house. My lovely breast-care nurses and the Breast Cancer Support Group donated some money so I could go for a short break to Bournemouth. Lisa and I set off on the train for a great couple of days in the sun. I love Bournemouth. It's my favourite place in the UK.

19 August 2006

I felt strange. There I was at the end of my treatment, but I thought, 'Hoo-*bloomin'*-ray!' At this time I felt my loneliest and most vulnerable. *Lost* is the word. I felt lost because I was now on my own with no more safety net of nurses and doctors and no more chemotherapy in my body to kill any lurking cancer cells. I wanted to live, but I was scared to plan my life when for the previous eight months I had been preparing for my death.

Recently somebody asked the question "Where do you see yourself in five years' time?"

ALIVE.

The Birth of Angel, 26—27 August 2006

I was supposed to go and see *Chitty Chitty Bang Bang* with Lisa – a treat given to us by my friend Cindy and her daughter Katie. Cindy and Katie had been friends of ours since our weekly visits to the Birmingham Hippodrome when Lisa was a junior associate and mid-associate in the Royal Ballet. However, I didn't get to see the show: Fiona went into early labour.

We stayed at home as long as she could cope with the contractions. Her pain strategy was to bite on a pillow. She coped really well, but I started to feel a little edgy about being at home, so off we went to the labour ward.

Fiona was a star. She was 5 cm dilated and halfway there. I was so excited. I thought, 'This is going well. It won't belong before I see my granddaughter. I couldn't wait. Nanny La La, was there in the background supporting us both.

As things were going so well, and because two people could be at the birth, Fiona agreed for Nanny La La to be the second birthing partner – three generations in the labour ward, waiting patiently for the arrival of our special gift, Angel.

Nanny La La got her name because one day she asked Jill and I if we were line dancing at the La La Bar? We laughed, and I said, "No, we are dancing salsa at the Ha Ha bar.

Things didn't quite work out as planned. How Nanny La La didn't have another one of her minor strokes I don't know! The birthing-partner experience was a complete nightmare. For nearly twenty-four hours Fiona suffered pain after pain. Her cervix would not dilate any further. In the end, they decided she needed an epidural. I hung on to Fiona for dear life as the anaesthetist said, "It's is dangerous if she moves when I am doing this procedure."

I felt helpless, seeing her in such pain, and I was beginning to get frightened. I had been a midwife for seven years, but that did nothing to reassure me. I knew too much. When it finally came to Fiona giving birth, I was a wreck. I will never forget the moment Angel's heart rate started to fall. I was moved out of the way and I watched in a trance as my poor daughter was mutilated with instruments – first the vacuum extraction equipment and then forceps. There were DRS and resuscitation trolleys in the room. I looked out of the window because I wanted to run out of the room, but I couldn't get past all the mayhem. There was no way I could bear to be in the room to hear the last heartbeat of my grandchild. I sobbed and sobbed and prayed and prayed: "Please, God, for once I've had enough. Do not take this gift from me, and do not take this gift from my daughter. Don't you dare!"

At last Angel was born, and to break the trauma Nanny La La shouted, "It's a boy!"

I said, "No it's not, Mum; it's a girl."

I ran over to the paediatrician and, as soon as she said she was all right, I shouted, "Give me that baby." I just looked at the miracle in my arms and cried. I cried eight months of tears in those few seconds.

I wished I hadn't turned around to look at Fiona, because I was faced with the aftermath of the birth, and Fiona was taken into theatre to repair the damage sustained from the delivery.

My gift, Erica Lisa Angel Gilbert, my first grandchild, was born – the birth of Angel!

"Nothing's gonna harm you, not while I'm around."
(Barbra Streisand)

Erica's birth was a turning point in my relationship with my ex-husband. Our mutual pride and love for our child and our grandchild erased oh, too many years of acrimonious separation, and that was very positive for our children and for us.

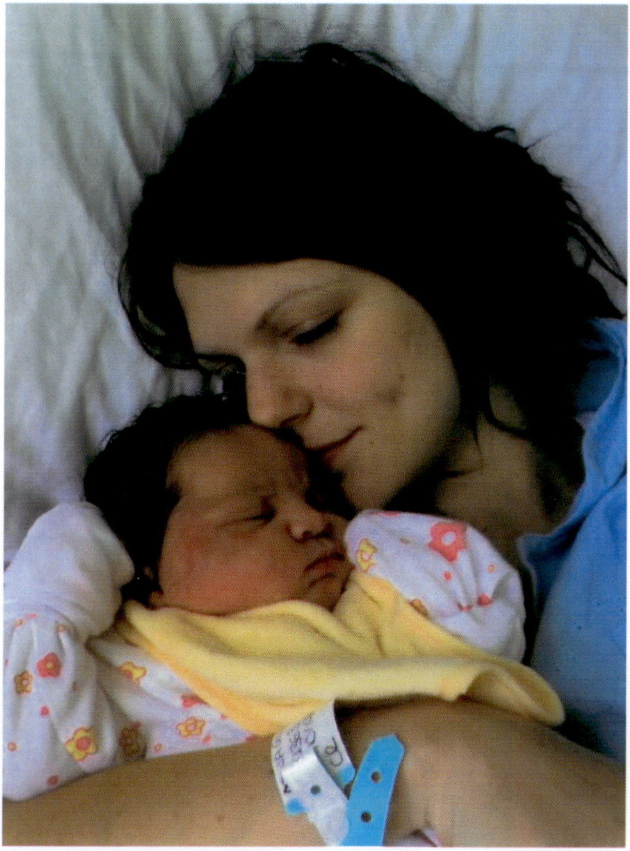

Fiona and Erica.

26 September 2006

I hadn't written in my journal lately because I had so much to say and couldn't put anything into words. I was not so bright and breezy and my legs hurt (apparently a side effect from withdrawal of the steroids) but I hoped to lose the appearance of a sumo wrestler, and my hair was growing back – short, black curly hair.

Negativity was engulfing me. I thought every little pain was the big C. I felt isolated. I missed the women in the chemo club, and the volunteers who had had breast cancer themselves and had lived to tell the tale and show us how good reconstructive surgery is. I had a friend with terminal cancer, and we shared some stories, but we couldn't share them all and, besides, I didn't want to. It was too painful.

The wonderful breast-care nurses organised a meeting of people who had just finished their treatment. The atmosphere in that meeting was one of mutual empathy. Every one of us was venturing on a new life. My previous life had ended eight months before. We all felt tearful, vulnerable and emotionally unstable, and we all had aching joints. We all cried when we mentioned our children.

From a singleton's point of view, I was interested to hear that the married women had also felt alone, as their husbands were as traumatised as they themselves were.

I shed many tears around this time.

29 September 2006

Indifferent is the word. I felt neither here nor there, on a plateau of emotion. I was simply not bothered.

There had been occasions when I thought being with my husband would have been easier. I was so bored with being single and alone, but I didn't want to play single predatory games any more.

Survives Cancer, Nearly Dies of Facial, 22 October 2006

My work colleagues had collected money and paid for me to join them at a very exclusive health spa. Before receiving a facial treatment I did speak to the nurse about my recent cancer treatment, but for some reason I had an allergic reaction to whatever was rubbed into my face and neck. I ended up whizzing off to the hospital in an ambulance.

November 2006

A month after the facial, I joined a walking party in the Lake District.

I didn't walk but sat in a coffee shop in Bowness-on-Windermere wondering if people really did look at the scenery as I did. Everything seemed so much more beautiful now – the beauty of the seasons, the snow on the mountain tops.

I am a very sociable person, but sometimes I like being alone to ponder and people-watch. I sometimes feel like an alien from 'cancer planet' – a person who visits normality only occasionally. When friends start talking about plans for the future, I drop out of the conversation. Planning special occasions – looking too far ahead – is now a thing of the past.

Oh dear! I ended up in the Southport hospital following a similar experience to the one at the health spa, but I survived to live another day.

Dating Again

Dating was to become interesting. If I mentioned breast cancer to men, some pretended to be good about it, some ran a mile, and some were upfront and told me that they could never deal with something like that. But, in a positive frame of mind, I returned to dating, and there was no real change in the dating game either good or bad, emotionally or sexually. I think this is a very positive lesson for fellow breast-cancer survivors: breast cancer makes no difference to your luck in love. You still have to deal with hurt and rejection.

I did meet somebody on 23 December 2006 and it was partly thanks to him that Christmas and New Year were memorable.

I was happy and I wondered if my luck was changing. Maybe, maybe not!

Christmas Day, 2006

Did we laugh! Fiona, Erica Lisa Angel, Lisa and Ali sat round the table with me. I had forgotten Christmas crackers. We had no wine so we drank Coca-Cola from the cans. None of us had got dressed. As we looked around the table at each other we burst out laughing, and at that moment all the cards fell off the wall.

Here we were, united as a family, happy, laughing, hopeful, celebrating family life.

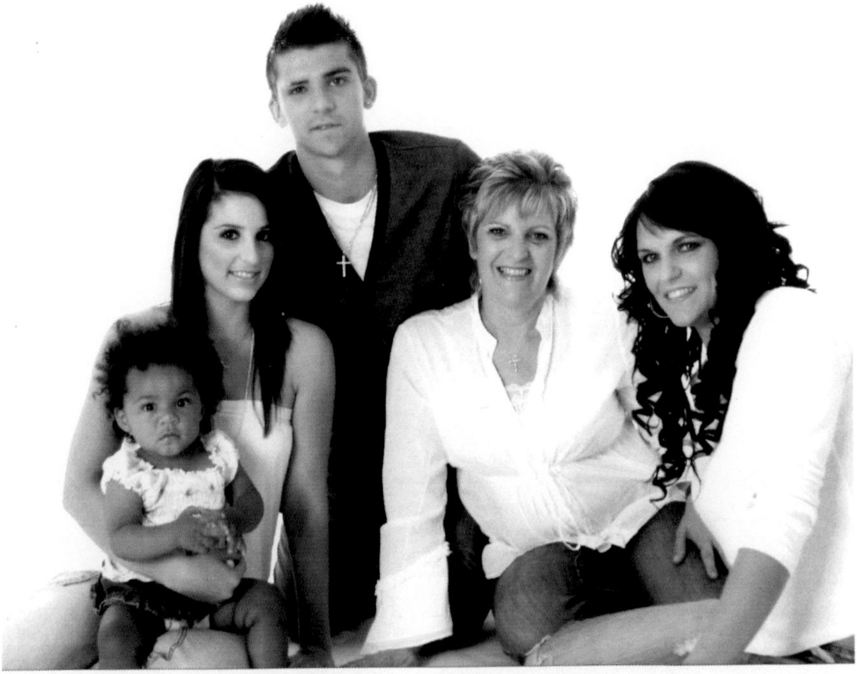

A year after treatment, with my family.

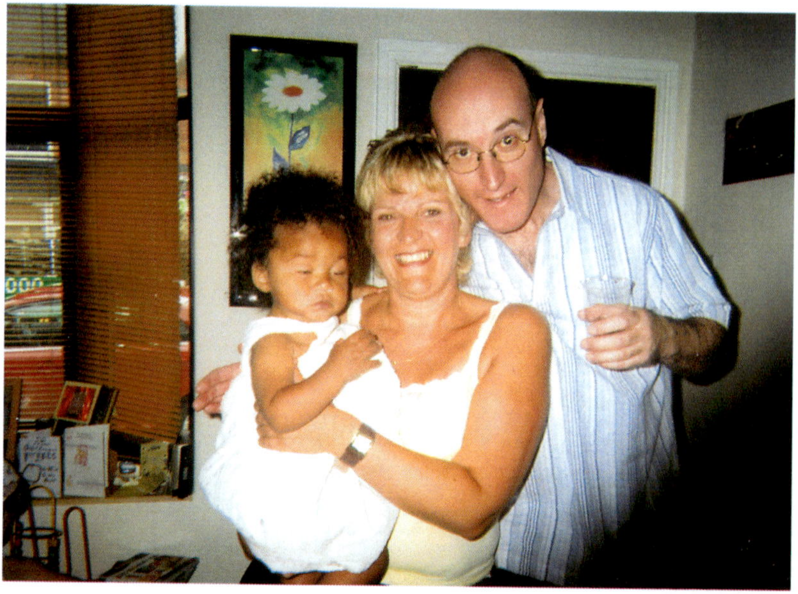

Erica's first birthday, August 2007.
My knight in shining armour, Graham.

Here to see another girly holiday, Magaluf, 2007.

Depression, December 2007

I entered the bubble of sadness where only I can go. Sometimes I peeped into the sunshine only to be knocked back into the sadness bubble by Mr Rejection, Miss No-Insight or Master Virus or just because I had grown comfortable in sadness.

No one could pull me out, and I kept slipping down as I tried to cling to the wall of gloom. I was in a black hole.

I needed counselling and I asked for professional help.

ME

What shall I do?
Where shall I go?
Who shall I be?
Will somebody see
I am no longer me?
From today I stay silent and create my own world –
A world where even my imagination is empty.

My soul is like ice, frozen solid and cold.
Only the times with Erica and my children
Melt a small corner of my solid soul.
What shall I do?
Where shall I go?
Who shall I be?
Will somebody see
I am no longer **ME**?

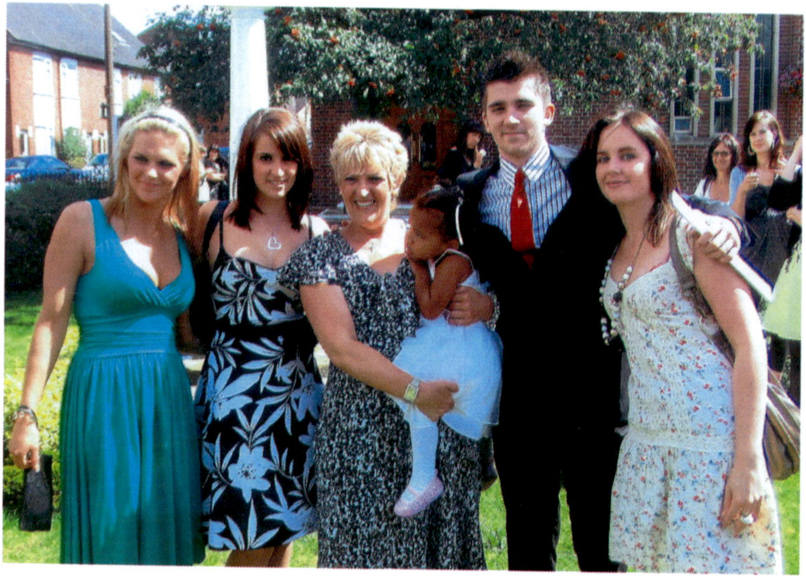

Happier times again, Erica's christening, August 2008.

Christmas Day 2008

I was supposed to be getting engaged today, *supposed* being the operative word: he just didn't turn up.

I have had so many life experiences since the cancer in 2005, and all of them have challenged my emotional stamina. Life carries on with its ups and downs. I had hoped I would only be granted the ups in life now that I had faced death.

Wrong! While I am still on this earth, life's challenges keep coming. I am responsible for my own destiny.

Life is about sunny days and happy memories.

We come into the world alone, and we may leave the world alone. It is what we do and who we meet in between that counts.

February 2009

I sat in the X-ray department at the local hospital. Mum was sitting, as per usual, in the waiting area. Both of us had been catapulted back to 2005 – déjà vu. I remembered the feeling in the waiting room three and a half years before. This time nobody averted their gaze; there was a feeling of normality and an aura of everyday business just happening as usual.

"The results are normal."

Thank goodness! A big sigh of relief!

25 February 2009

Tragedy struck our family. I can't speak about this yet.

7 March 2009

I met Chris.

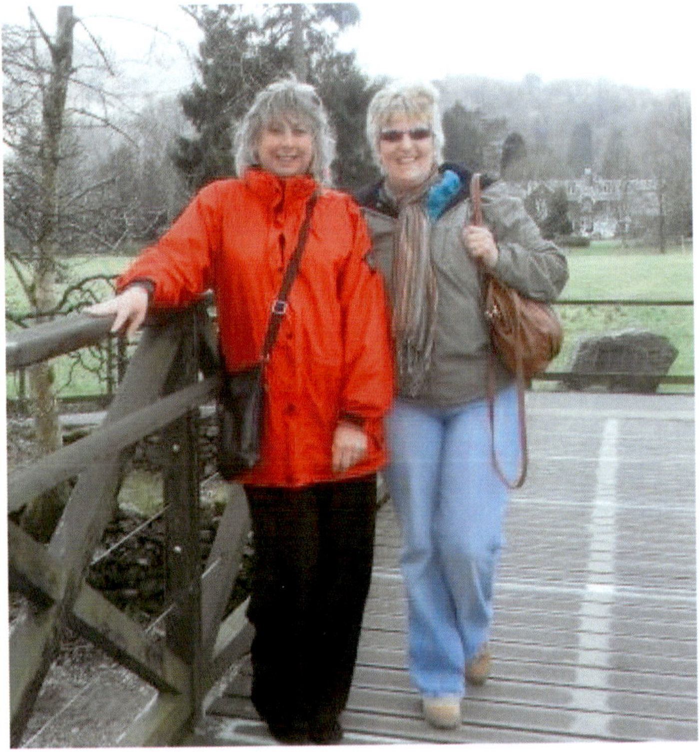

Me and my best friend, Janine, celebrating our fiftieth birthdays a year early, at Grasmere, in the Lake District, March 2009.

Gran Canaria, 28 April to 4 May 2009

I lie on golden sands surrounded by dramatic volcanic rock. My favourite crimson flowers cover the white walls of the hotels and holiday homes. Beach cafés line the harbour. This is real – neither a dream nor a fantasy.

I suddenly feel at ease, revelling in happiness with my new man, Chris. I remember what it was like to embrace the fantastic experiences of life and I believe I have a future again. Past life experiences float out to sea.

Cancer may land again on my shore and it may not, but until then I *'embrace uncertainty'*. (Susan Jeffers)

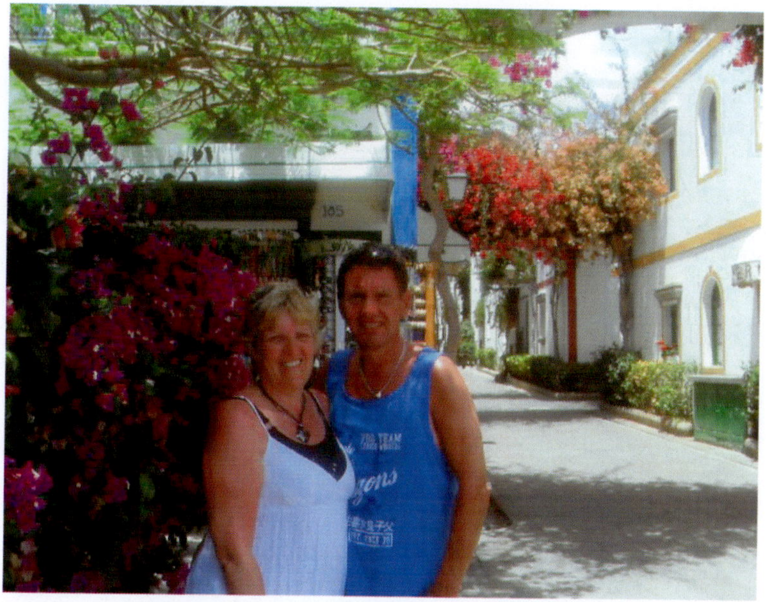

With Chris, Gran Canaria, April 2009.

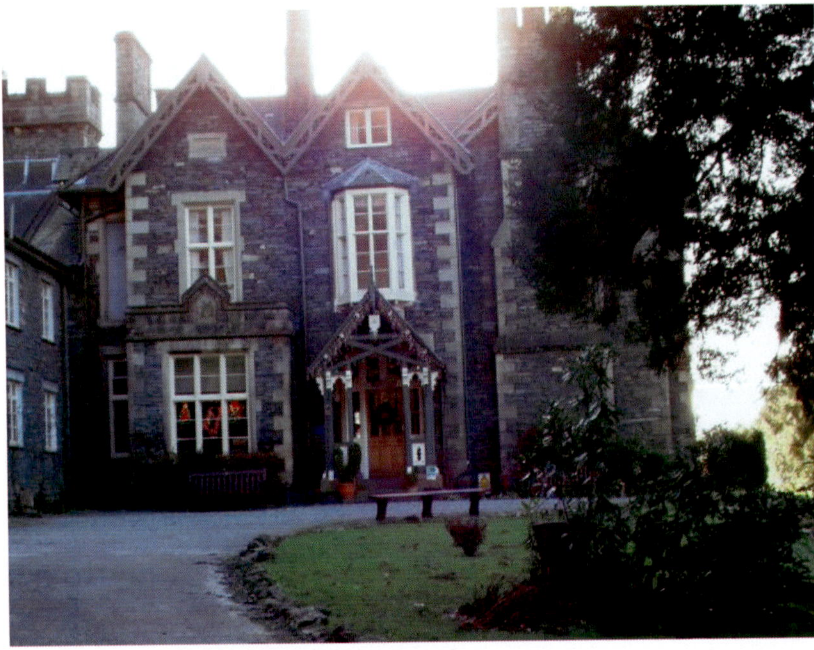

Forest Side Hotel, Grasmere,
where I typed my journal, October 2007.

Not the end, but just the beginning.